TABLE OF CONTENTS

INTRODUCTION

Your heart is the major organ of your cardiovascular system, a network of blood vessels that pumps blood throughout your body. It also works with other body systems to control your heart rate and blood pressure. Your family history, personal health history and lifestyle all affect how well your heart works.The heart beats about 2.5 billion times over the average lifetime, pushing millions of gallons of blood to every part of the body. When the heart stops, essential functions fail, some almost instantly.

A healthy lifestyle goes a long way to preventing cardiovascular disease.In this book I will be creating more insight on the heart(structure and functions),heart attack&Cardiac arrest,CPR, 10 healthy foods for the heart,foods to avoid and a healthy lifestyle to promote your heart health.

The Heart

The heart is a muscular fist-sized

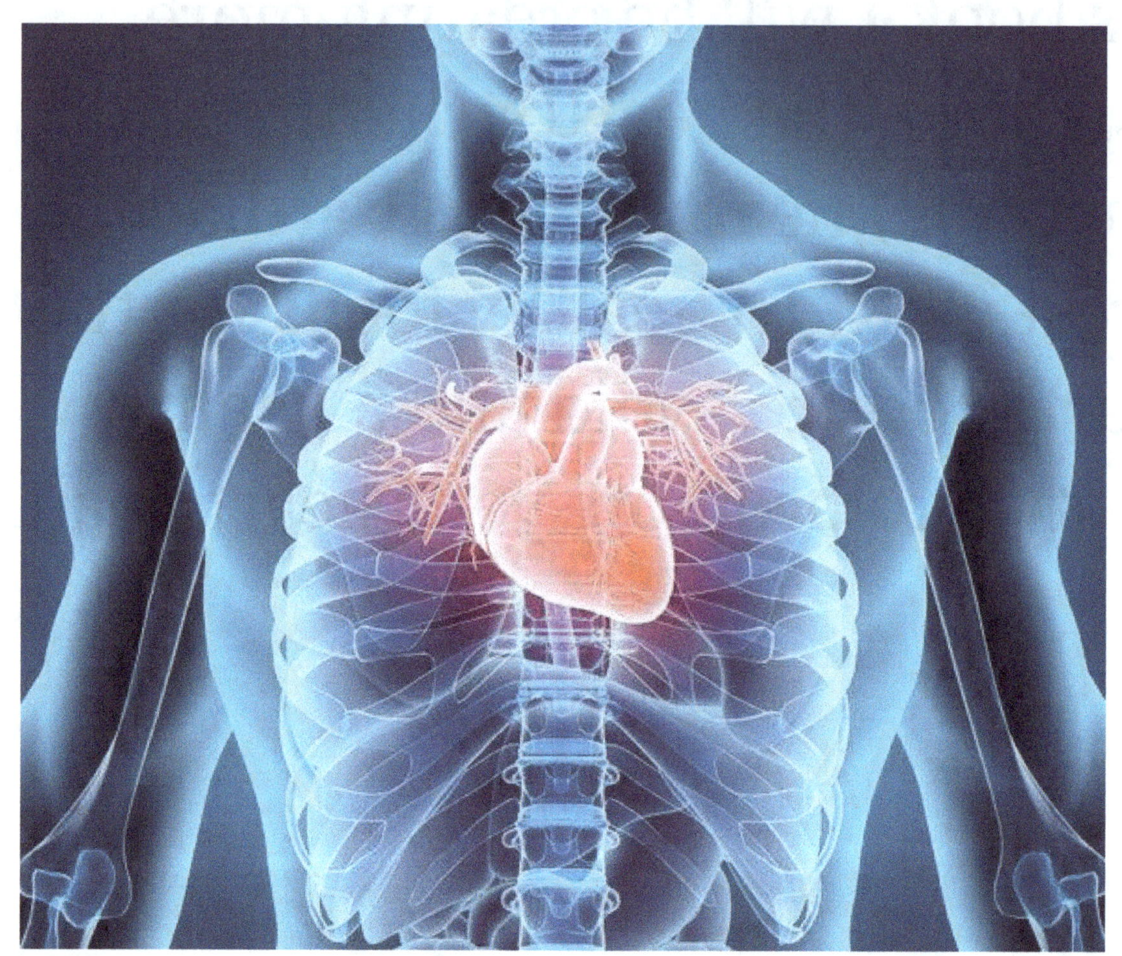

organ(meaning the heart is the size of an Adult

fist),situated in the chest just behind and slightly toward the left of the breastbone.

It's the primary organ of the cardiovascular/circulatory System.

The heart works all the time, pumping blood through the network of blood vessels called the arteries and veins.

The heart, blood and its blood vessels are known as the cardiovascular system.

The heart contains four main sections (chambers) made of muscle and powered by electrical impulses.

The brain and nervous system direct your heart's function.

Chambers of the Heart

The internal cavity of the heart is

divided into four chambers:

- Right atrium
- Right ventricle
- Left atrium
- Left ventricle

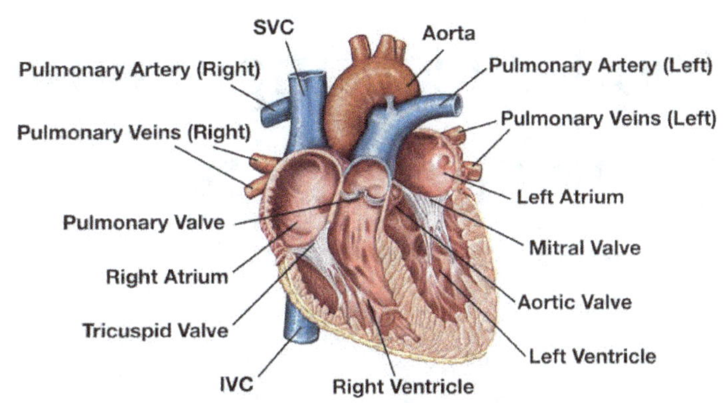

The two atria are thin-walled chambers receive blood from the veins. The right atrium receives deoxygenated blood from systemic veins; the left atrium receives oxygenated blood from the pulmonary veins.

The two ventricles are thick-walled chambers that forcefully pump blood out of the heart.Atria are thin and have less muscular walls and are smaller than ventricles. These are the blood-receiving chambers that are fed by the large veins.

Ventricles are larger and more muscular chambers responsible for pumping and pushing blood out into circulation.These are connected to larger arteries that deliver blood for circulation.

On the right side of the heart,The right atrium and ventricle work to pump oxygen-poor blood to the lungs. On the left side, the left atrium and ventricle combine to pump oxygenated blood to the body.

Three layers of tissue form the heart wall. The outer layer of the heart wall is the *epicardium,* the middle layer is the *myocardium,* and the inner layer is the *endocardium.*

Blood Vessels

In the human body, blood flows within vessels of varying sizes.The external structure of the heart has many blood vessels that form a network, with other major vessels emerging from within the structure.

3 Types of blood vessels

Veins :Veins are blood vessels that carries blood back to the heart.it supplies deoxygenated blood to the heart via inferior and superior vena cava.

Arteries:Arteries are blood vessels that carries blood away from the heart.They are muscular-walled tube that carries oxygenated blood away from the heart to all other parts of the body. *Aorta* is the largest of the arteries and it branches off into various smaller arteries throughout the body.

Capillaries

 Capillaries are the smallest blood vessels that connects arteries to veins.They are tiny, tube-like vessels which form a network between the arteries to veins.

The heart pumps around 6,000-7,500 litres of blood in a day throughout the body.

Functions of the Heart

1.Its significant role is to pump blood throughout the body

2.Enables transport of oxygen-rich blood to all components of the body.

3.Helps regulate adequate/maintaining blood pressure throughout the body.

4.Transfers nutrients to cells, tissues, and all parts of the body.

5.Circulating hormones and other essential substances to different parts of the body.

6.Removing metabolic waste such as carbon dioxide from all the tissues in the body.

Some Heart Facts:

•The heart pumps around 6,000-7,500 litres of blood in a day throughout the body.

•The heart is situated at the centre o f the chest and points slightly towards the left.

•On average, the heart beats about 100,000 times a day, i.e., around 3 billion beats in a lifetime.

•The average male heart weighs around 280 to 340 grams (10 to 12 ounces). In females, it weighs around 230 to 280 grams (8 to 10 ounces).

•An adult's heart beats about 60 to 100 times per minute, and a newborn baby's heart beats at a faster pace than an adult which is about 90 to 190 beats per minute.

•Other than the cornea, every cell in the human body gets blood from the heart.

•The average heart is the size of a fist in an adult.

•Normal Blood pressure is considered to be within 90/60mmHg and 120/80mmHg. high blood pressure is considered to be 140/90mmHg or higher.

- Pulse rate=60-100 beats/min.

10 MOST AMAZING FOODS FOR A HEALTHY HEART.

1.Avocado: Avocado is an excellent source of heart-healthy monounsaturated fats, which have been linked to reduced levels of cholesterol and a lower risk of heart disease.avocadoes helps in reducing

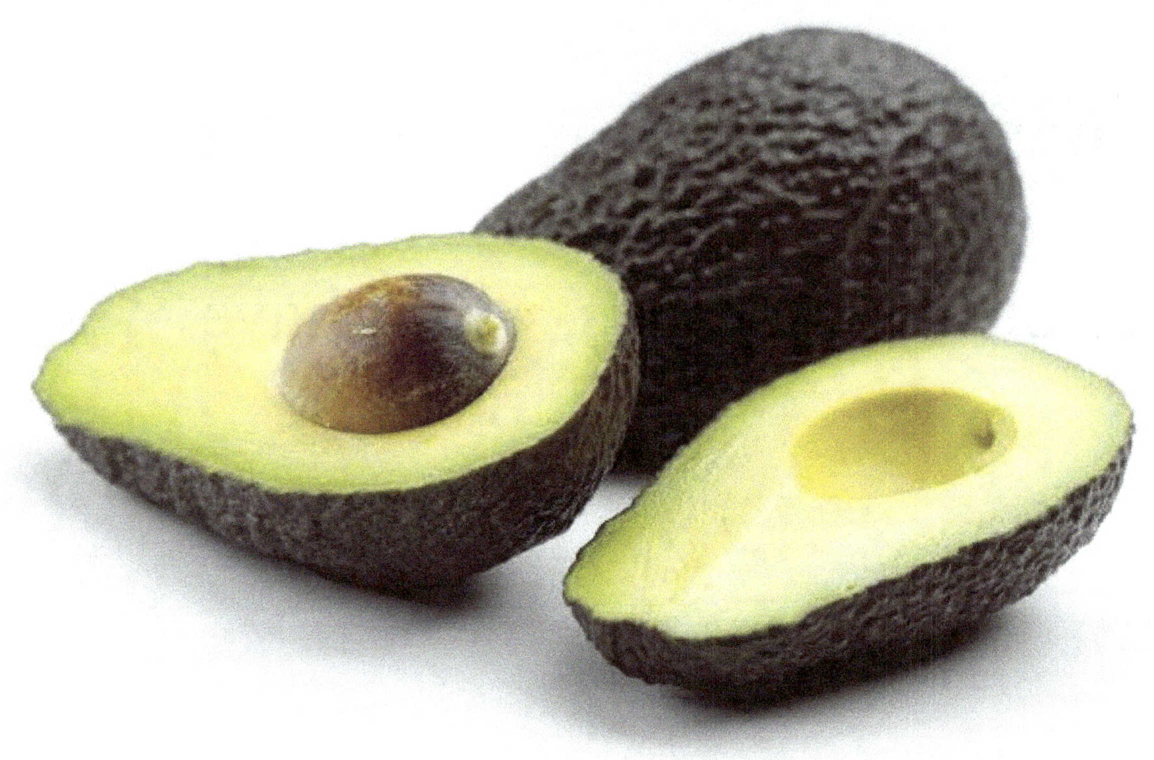

LDL (bad) cholesterol, including

lower levels of small, dense LDL (bad)

cholesterol, which is believed to raise

the risk of heart disease.

 Avacodoes possess a lipid-lowering and cardioprotective benefit.

Avocados are also rich in potassium, a nutrient that's essential to heart health.

2. Whole grains:

Whole grains include all three nutrient-rich parts of the grain:germ

Endosperm bran.

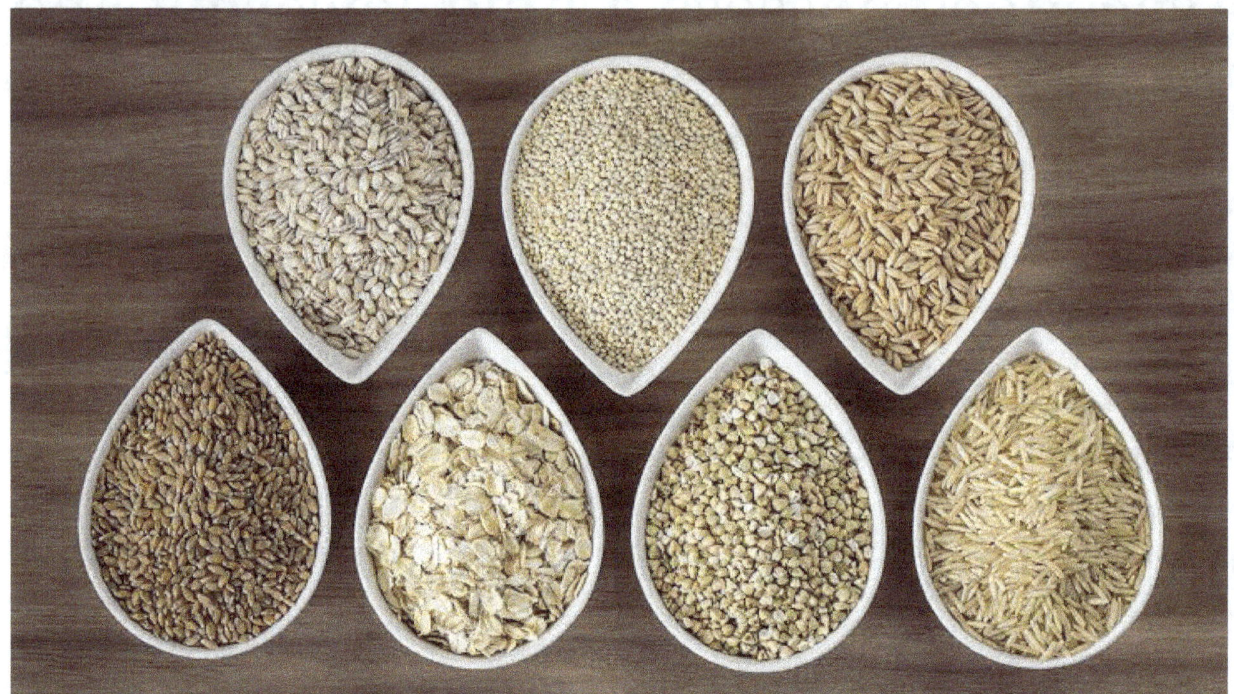

Common types of whole grains include:

whole wheat

brown rice

oats

rye

barley

Millet

quinoa

Refined carbohydrates increase the risk of coronary heart disease. Conversely, whole grains are protective.

Multiple studies have found that including more whole grains in your diet can benefit your heart health.

Adopting a diet rich in plant-based foods, whole grains, low fat dairy products, and sodium intake within normal limits can be effective in the prevention and management of hypertension.Studies show that eating whole grains is associated with lower cholesterol and systolic blood pressure, as well as a lower risk of heart disease.

3.Fatty fish and fish oil

Fatty fish like salmon, mackerel, sardines, and tuna are loaded with omega-3 fatty acids, which have been studied extensively for their heart-health benefits.

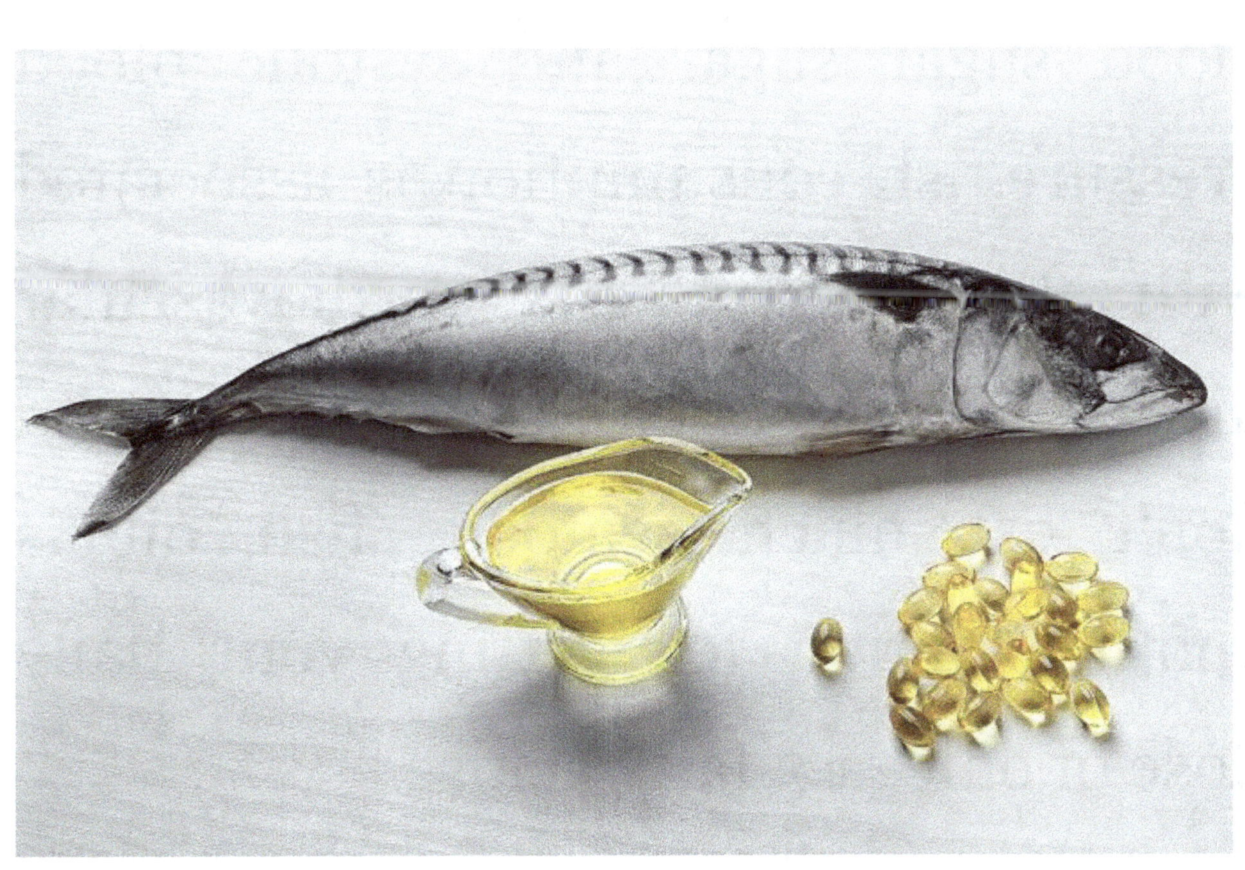

Omega-3 fatty acids from fatty fish may have a protective role in the risk of developing heart disease.

Eating fish over the long term was linked to lower levels of total cholesterol, blood triglycerides, fasting blood sugar sugar and systolic blood pressure.fish consumption is associated with lower risk of Cardiovascular disease, depression and mortality.If you don't eat much seafood, fish oil is another option for getting your daily dose of omega-3 fatty acids.

Other omega-3 supplements like krill oil or algal oil are popular alternatives.

Fatty fish and fish oil are both high in omega-3 fatty acids and may help reduce heart disease risk factors, including blood pressure, triglycerides, and cholesterol.

4.Almonds: Almonds are incredibly nutrient-dense, boasting a long list of vitamins , minerals that are crucial to

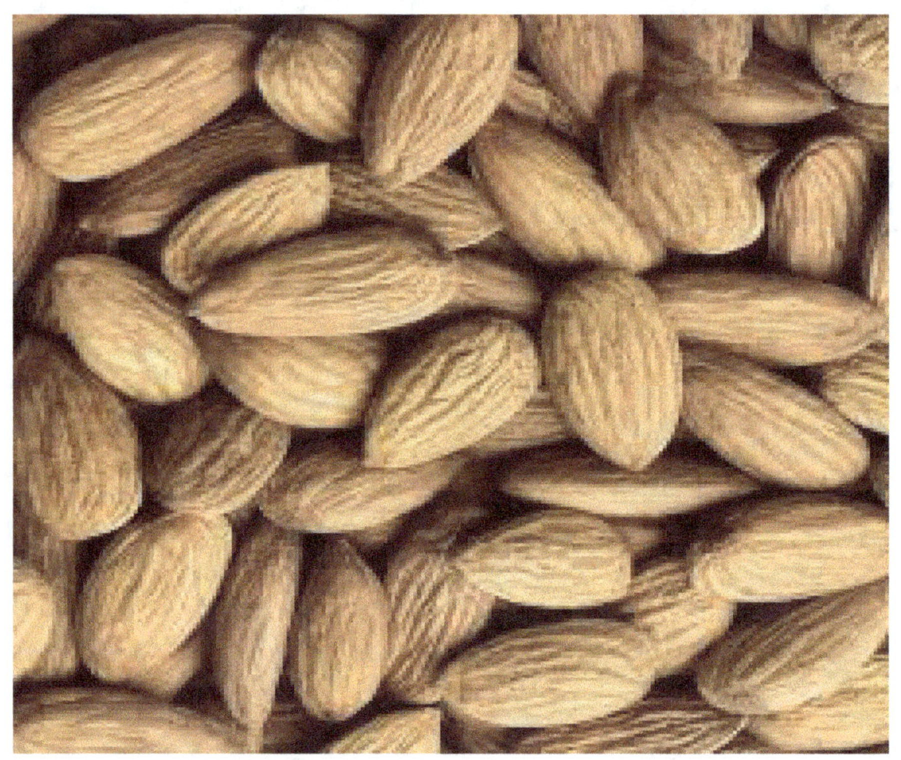

heart health.

They're also a good source of heart-healthy monounsaturated fats and fiber, two important nutrients that can help protect against heart disease.

Almonds consumption can have a powerful effect on your cholesterol levels.almonds are associated with higher levels of HDL (good) cholesterol, which can help reduce plaque buildup and keep your arteries clear.Remember that while almonds are very high in nutrients, they're also high in calories. Measure your portions and moderate your intake if you're trying to lose weight.They are high in fiber and monounsaturated fats, and have been linked to reductions in cholesterol and belly fat.

5.Green Tea:Green tea has been associated with a number of health benefits, from increased fat burning to improved insulin sensitivity.It contains

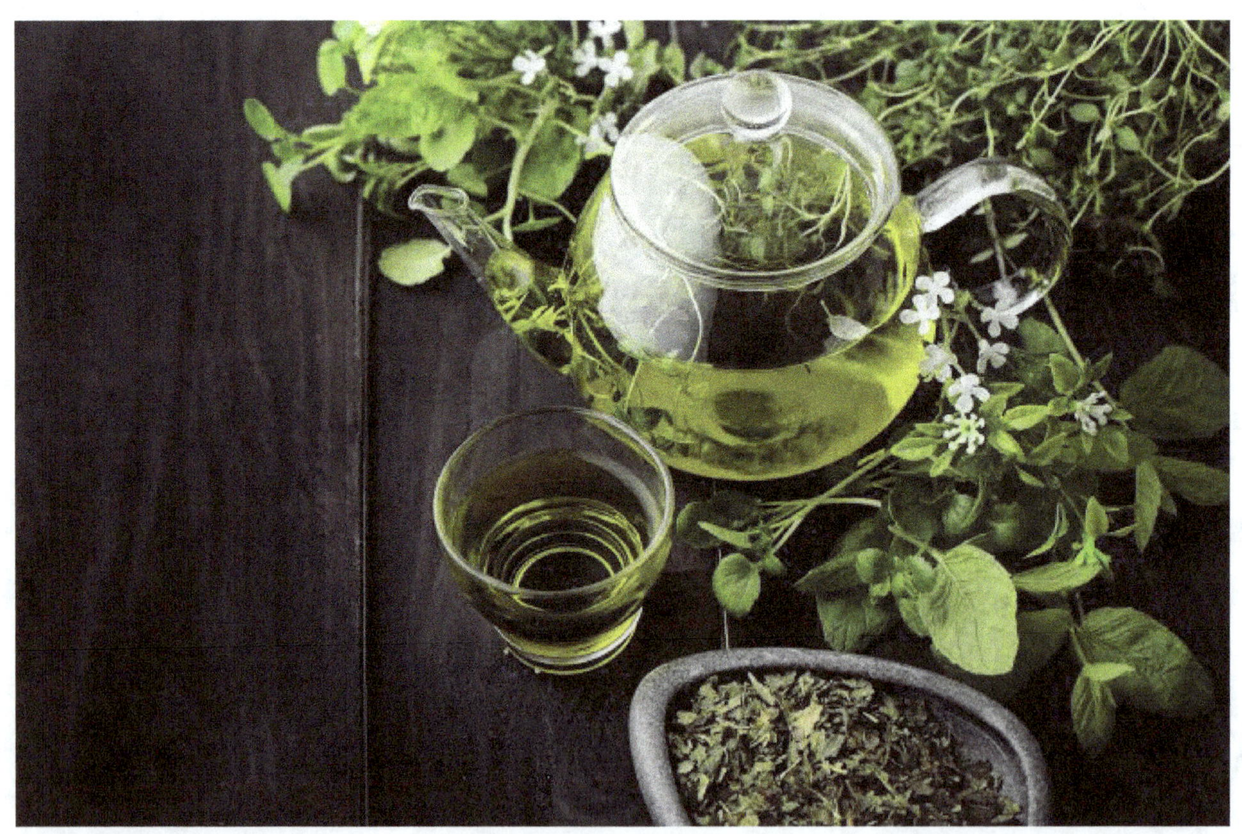

polyphenols and catechins, which can

act as antioxidants to prevent cell damage, reduce inflammation, and protect the health of your heart.

6.Berries: Berries have been described as "superfruits" as they are capable of blocking as well as reversing most of the aging consequences. They are incredible

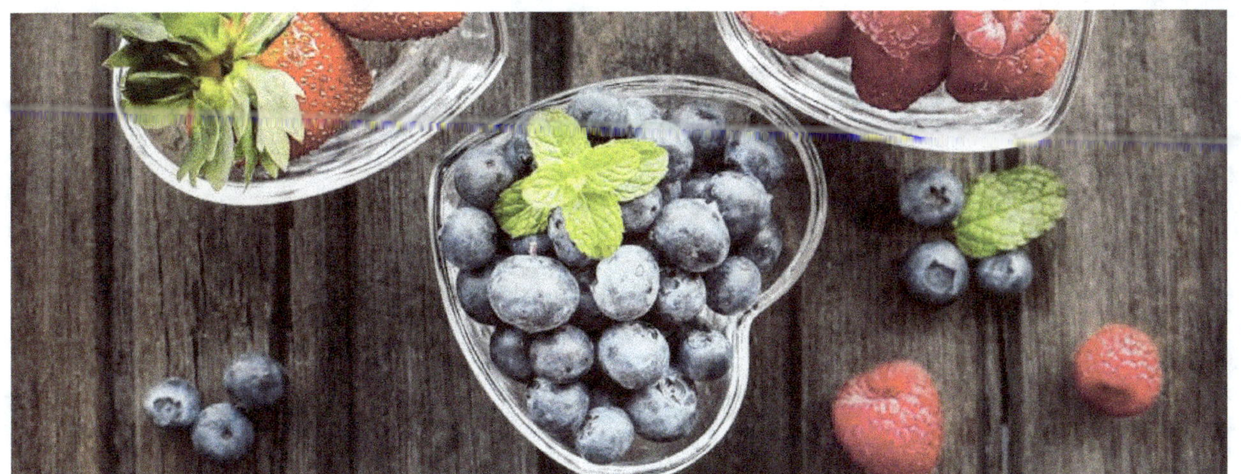

anti-aging food that keeps the brain healthy by boosting mental health. The dark hues present in berries shows their high antioxidant content, which ward off free radicals that lead to aging and helps Us to stay healthy.

Besides being a powerhouse sources of antioxidants which delivers multiple benefits,berries also possess the abilities to bring positive impacts to multiple aging processes. Recent studies have shown that blueberry extracts can significantly increase life span. Blueberries also deliver maximum nutrition for minimum calories. With regular consumption, belly fat could also be reduced.

In comparison to other fruits, blueberries contain less sugar so it is less likely to affect your insulin levels, making them a great option for a fast guiltless snack. As they are low-glycemic fruits, they help to keep your insulin levels balanced as well as keep you focused. These fruits are also packed with fiber which keeps your digestion on track, maintain your cholestrol levels, and develop a healthy weight necessary for optimal longevity.

Berries of all kinds are healthy which contain concentrated amounts of phytochemicals which help to fight heart disease, DNA damage, metabolic syndrome and even cancer. As a result, blood vessels will be more flexible which can help avoid the risks of developing a heart disease. Rather than the whole fruit, it's the particular flavonoid components of blueberries which deliver so many healthy benefits. These compounds are able to enhance high blood pressure, decrease cardiovascular risk factors as well as enable the brain to function well even after stroke. Recent studies have proven that blueberries help to prevent brain deterioration as well as protect memory-associated regions of the brain from possible oxidant and inflammatory damages.

Blueberries are becoming a critical element of a science-based longevity program due to their richness in anthocyanins and pterostilbenes.

Researches have discovered new data showing that blueberries are capable of delaying aging and can lead to longevity.

7.Dark Chocolate (Cocoa and Cocoapowder

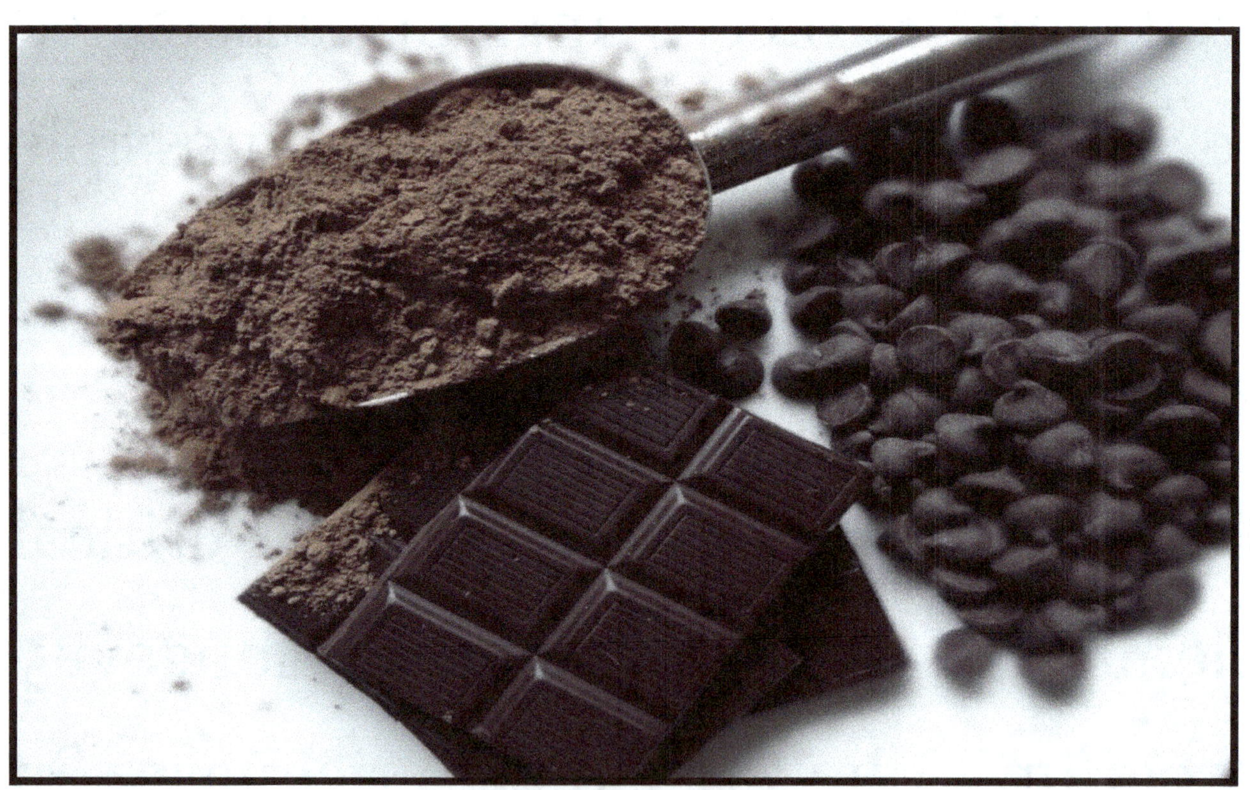

Research has shown that the indulgent of dark chocolate leads to more than 40 distinct nutrition benefits which includes longevity. Dark chocolate is an excellent source of antioxidants in the world which is made from the seed of the cocoa tree. It is most effective when cocoa or chocolate is eaten when it is raw (cacao) because when your cocoa is close to or in its natural raw state, they contain the highest nutritional value. In fact, Cacao is one of the most beneficial foods that helps to facilitate a healthy heart and brain. Moreover, cacao aids in lowering blood sugar, blood pressure, and its healthy fats are actually beneficial for your body compared to animal-based saturated fats.

In reference to a 2007 paper found in Journal of Nutrition, dark chocolate is loaded with a group of antioxidants called flavonoids which have been proven to avoid cardiovascular disease. It also added that eating quality dark chocolate containing a high cocoa content is more beneficial, especially when there is 70 percent of cocoa or more. Both raw cacao and cocoa are wonderful [heart-healthy foods](#) which enhance hormones, circulation and even your digestion.

Basically, if you want to reward yourself with a sweet snack and maintain your health at the same time, dark chocolate may in fact be the best choice due to the various health benefits it offers. But, bear in mind that it is also rich in fat. Apart from keeping track of your fat intake, you may also opt for raw cacao powder or organic cocoa powder. Regular consumption of dark chocolate helps to break down bacteria and ferment its components into anti-inflammatory compounds which will benefit your overall health in the long run. Other than that, dark chocolate helps to prevent blood clots from forming and improve blood circulation.

Dark chocolate also acts as a mood booster as it contains some chemical compounds which exert a positive effect on your mind. It contains phenylethylamine (PEA), which allows your brain to release endorphins. So, consuming dark chocolate will help to brighten up your mood and makes you feel happier. A 1999 Harvard survey which consists of 8000 men has revealed that those who ate dark chocolate at least 3 times per month were able to live an extra year compared to those who didn't.

8.Leafy Greens and Green Vegetables

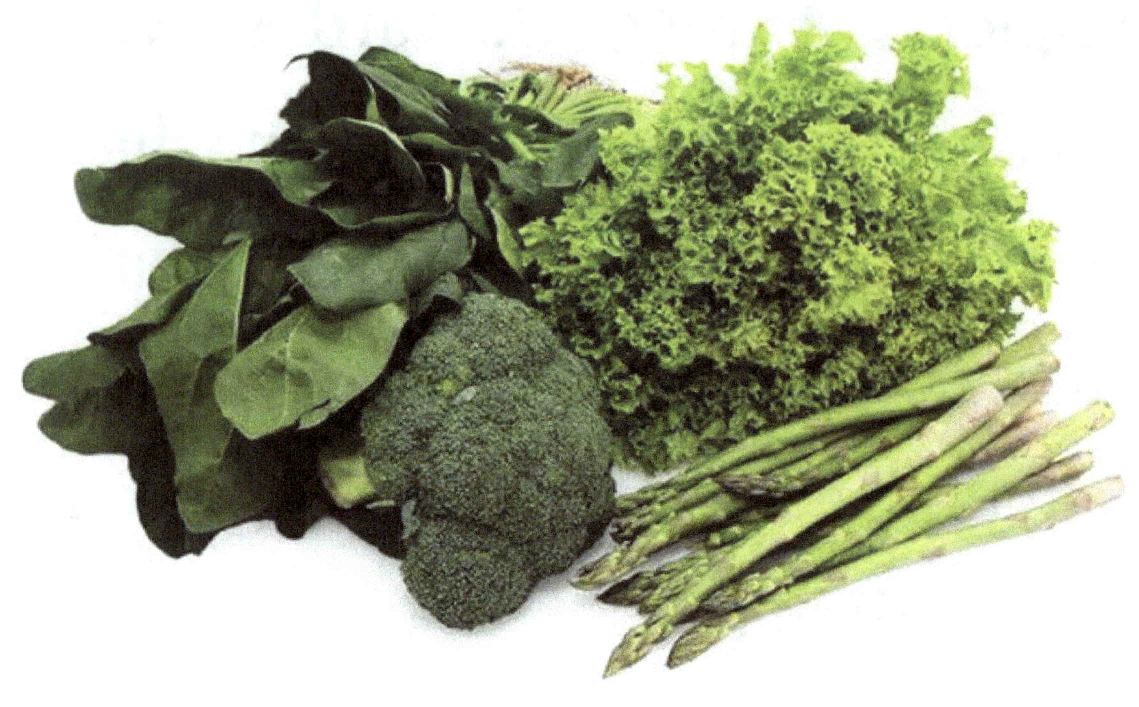

Green foods are heart-healthy foods and the key cornerstone of every healthy dietary living plan for optimal health. They're loaded with sufficient vitamins, protein, minerals and are known as the most alkaline-foods that can be found throughout the year. Leafy green vegetables such as broccoli, kale and spinach are few of the best to consume because they're rich in protein, calcium, magnesium, cholorophyll and irons.

Along with B6 vitamins, Vitamins A and C are also found in leafy green vegetables. Kale provides high vitamin K content for bone-building, which is necessary to stay active all year round. Leafy greens are also proven to be the best anti- cancer foods which play important roles in blocking the early phase of cancer and can even reverse the outcome of some major health problems. They are packed with an abundance of carotenoids-antioxidants and some other compounds which are created for protection against diseases. The antioxidants act as an agent in safeguarding the heart against cardiovascular disease and helps prevent some birth defects.

Moreover, the vitamin found in leafy green vegetables helps to reduce homocysteine levels which lowers the risk of heart disease. One of the most attractive benefits of dark leafy greens is that they contain low levels of calorie, carbohydrate and glycemic index. These characteristics allow them to facilitate maintaining and achieving the optimum healthy body weight. Including more green vegetables in a balanced diet causes an increase in dietary fiber intake which helps to regulate the digestive system, achieve bowel health as well as weight management.

Researchers have discovered that a gene known as T-bet respond particularly to leafy greens. These immune cells are vital for the production of immune cells present in your gut, responsible in handling inflammatory diseases and can even reduce the risk of bowel cancer. People who do not eat three or more servings of dark leafy greens per day are missing out on major health advantages.

Vegetables belong to a diverse food group with a wide variety to select from and plenty to match everyone's tastes and preferences. The easiest and most effective ways to increase vegetable intake is by juicing your vegetables with sprouted beans. This is because juicing makes it easily digestible and allows your body to absorb every nutrient present in the vegetables where some micronutrients may be lost during cooking. Based on a featured article, middle-aged people who eat a cup of cooked greens each day are able to live longer than those who didn't add leafy greens in their meal.

9.Red Wine and Resveratrol

If you drink alcohol, a little red wine may be a heart-healthy choice. [Resveratrol](#) and catechins, two antioxidants in red wine, may protect artery walls. Alcohol can also boost HDL, the good cholesterol.

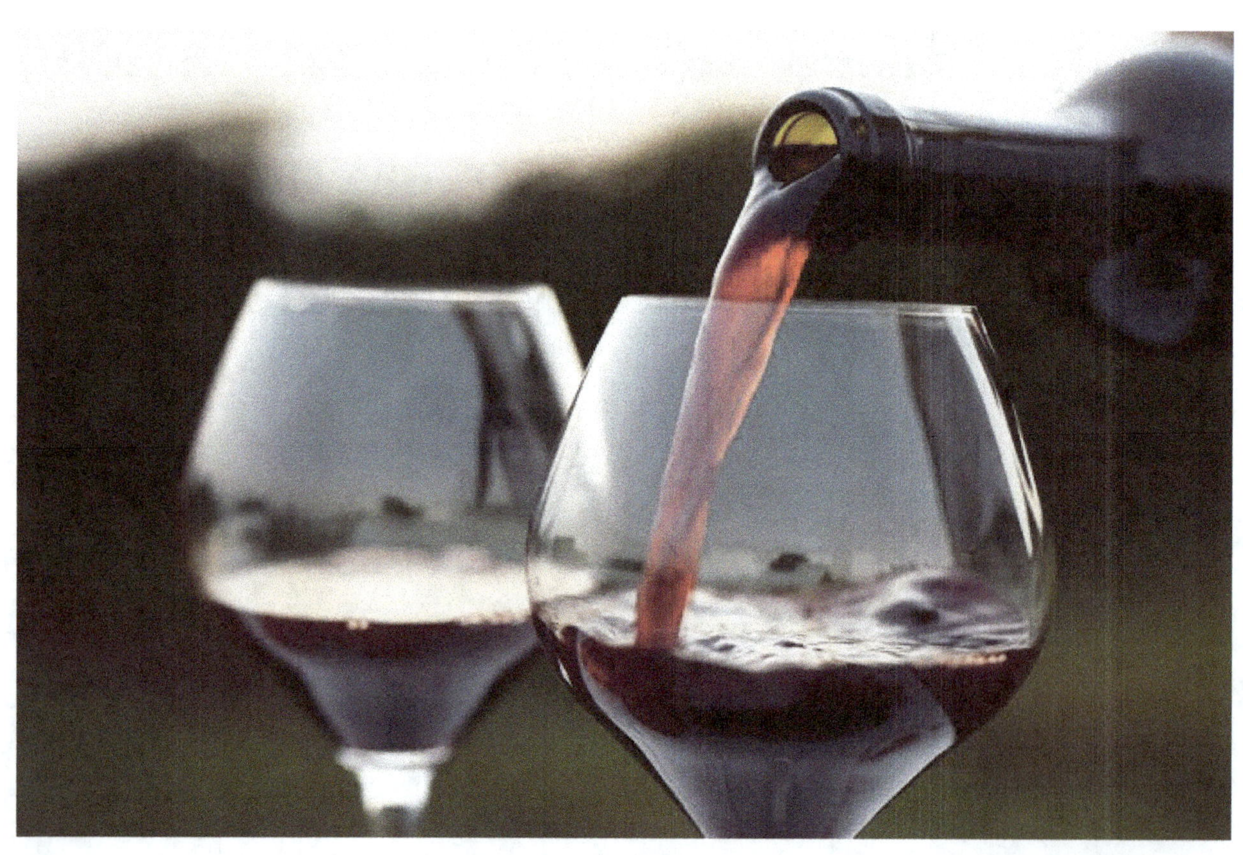

Tip: Too much alcohol hurts the heart. It's best to talk to your doctor first. Alcohol may cause problems for people taking aspirin and other medications.

10.Apples A group of research studies indicates that apples may be one of the world's healthiest fruits for you to include in your longevity diet plan.

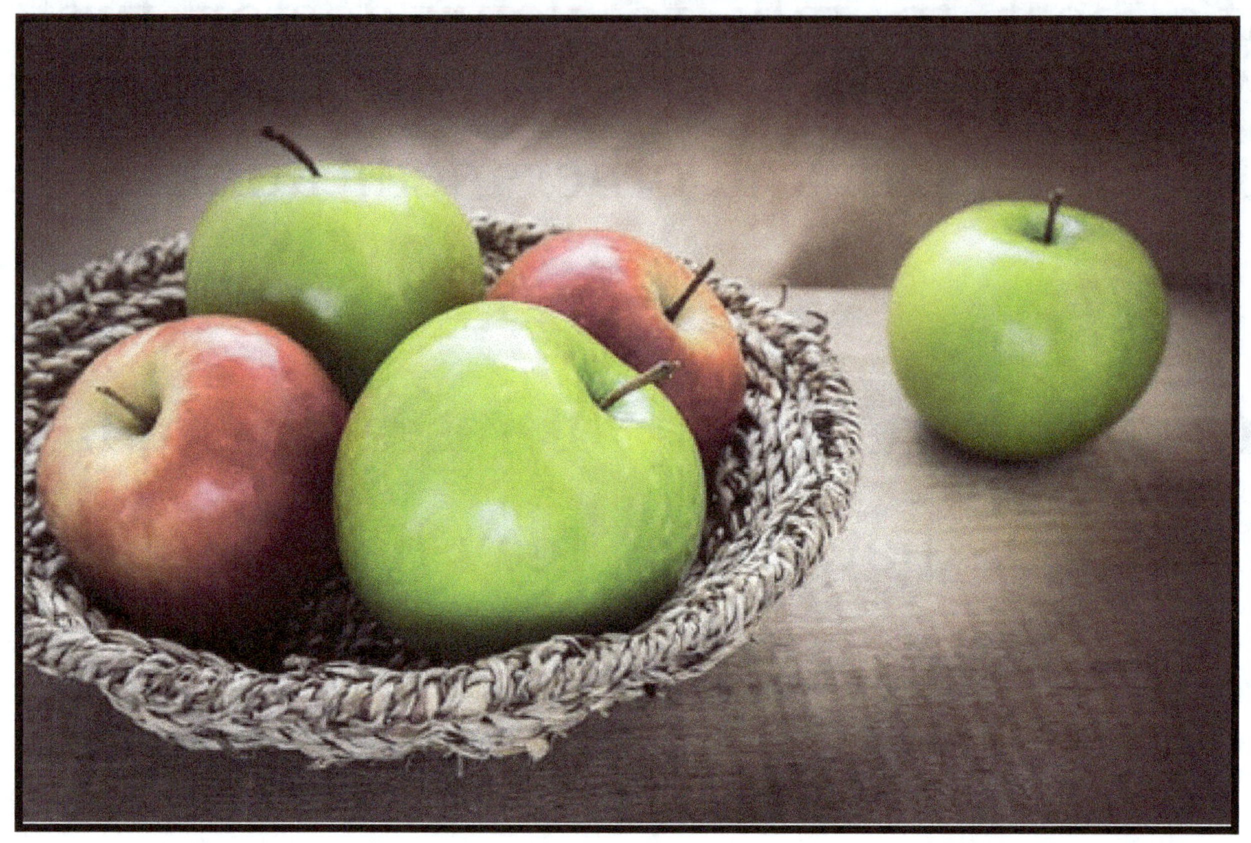

As they are the most commonly consumed fruit, people tend to overlook their impressive health benefits. In fact, in a featured article regarding the top 10 healthy foods in Medical News Today, apples were ranked first among the others. The old saying which we are all familiar with still stands true as an apple a day may be the ultimate food to promote longevity due to several health benefits it offers.

Firstly, apples are rich in vitamin C, fiber, various antioxidants and folate to fight against Alzheimer's. Moreover, they contain polyphenols which function as oxidants and are mainly concentrated in the peel. So, to achieve the greatest benefits, it is best to eat the apple's skin.These   polyphenols   contain flavonoids known as quercetin which helps to lower blood pressure. Studies have shown that high flavonoids intake have led to a 20% reduction in risk of stroke. Researchers agreed that consuming apples that are rich in flavonol could decrease the risk of getting pancreatic cancer by 23 percent.

By referring to Flores, it stated that regular apple consumption has been proven to provide cardiovascular benefits due to the fiber which they contain as well as the high contents of polyphenols found in apples. Flores also mentioned that the antioxidant level in apples has the highest rank compared to other fruits which help to prevent the risk of developing cancer, specifically lung cancer. Another study analyzes the comparison between the impacts of consuming an apple a day and statins which are a group of drugs taken to lower cholestrol level. It is estimated that apples are almost as effective as statins in minimizing death.

In a nut shell, apples contain several nutrients in a way which sets them apart from other fruits and makes them an excellent food choice for achieving good health in order to promote longevity.

FOODS TO AVOID

- Red meat.
- Bacon, hot dogs and other processed meats.
- French fries and other fried foods.
- Sugary drinks and cereals.
- Excess Salt(Sodium).
- Snack foods.
- Full-fat dairy products.
- Baked goods, cookies, and pastries
- Fatty and marbled meats.
- Spareribs.
- Fried or breaded meats.

Heart Attack and Cardiac Arrest.

Cardiac arrest is not the same as a heart attack but are all emergency cases.

A heart attack happens when blood flow to the heart is blocked. During a heart attack, an artery that sends blood and oxygen to the heart is blocked.

cholesterol &fatty deposits build up over time, forming plaques in the heart's arteries. If a plaque ruptures, a blood clot can form. The clot can block arteries, causing a heart attack.

This person *does not* need CPR—but they do need to get to
the hospital right away. Heart attack increases the risk for going into cardiac arrest.

Cardiac Arrest is when a person's heart stops beating. During cardiac arrest, the heart cannot pump blood to the rest of the body, including the brain and lungs. Death can happen in minutes without treatment. CPR uses chest compressions to mimic how the heart pumps. These compressions help keep blood flowing throughout the body.

CPR(Cardiopulmonary Resuscitation)-

CPR stands for Cardiopulmonary resuscitation. It can help save a life during cardiac arrest, when the heart stops beating or beats too ineffectively to circulate blood to the brain and other vital organs.As long

as a person having a heart attack is

alert and breathing, there is no need

for CPR. Cardiac arrest is not the

same as a heart attack. Someone whose heart has stopped beating is in cardiac arrest and needs CPR.CPR could be a lifesaver. Just remember to call emergency services before taking any action.

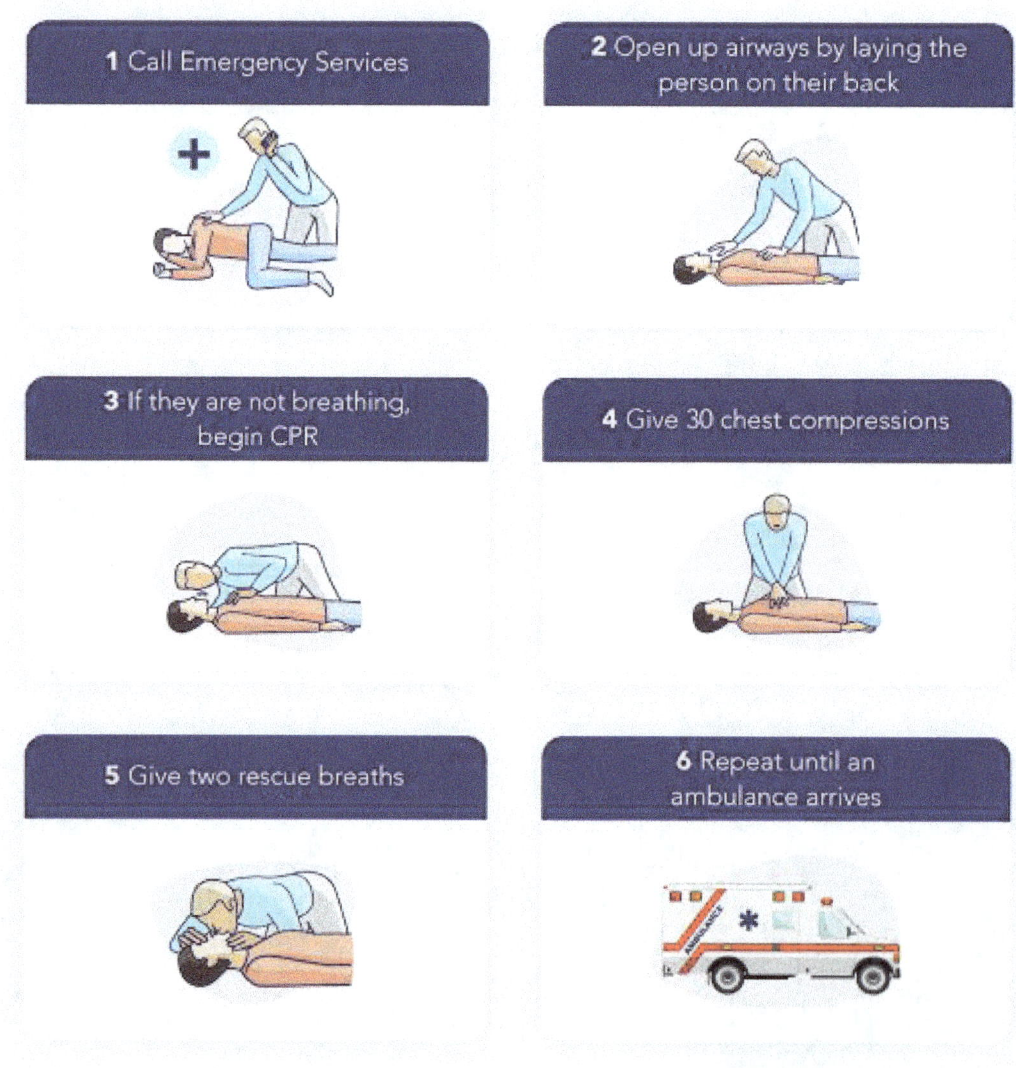

CPR step-by-step

•Call Emergency

•Check the scene for factors that could put you in danger, such as traffic, fire, or falling masonry.

•Kneel beside the person. Place the person on their back on a firm, flat surface.

•Open their airway and check for breathing.

•Perform 30 chest compressions. Here's how

Hand position:Intertwist both hands well centered on the chest

Body position: Shoulders directly over hands; elbows locked

Depth: At least 2 inches

Rate: 100 to 120 per minute

Allow chest to return to normal position after each compression

•Perform two rescue breaths. ...

-Open the airway to a past-neutral position using the head-tilt/chin-lift technique

-Pinch the nose shut, take a normal breath, and make complete seal over the person's mouth with your mouth.

-Ensure each breath lasts about 1 second and makes the chest rise; allow air to exit before giving the next breath

Note: If the 1st breath does not cause the chest to rise, retilt the head and ensure a proper seal before giving the 2nd breath If the 2nd breath does not make the chest rise, an object may be blocking the airway

•Continue giving sets of 30 chest compressions and 2 breaths until help arrives.

Causes of Heart Attack.

Coronary heart disease (CHD) is the leading cause of heart attacks. CHD is a condition in which the coronary arteries (the major blood vessels that supply the heart with blood) become clogged with deposits of cholesterol. These deposits are called plaques.

Diabetes and Cholesterol triggers heart attack.

Some **Unhealthy lifestyles** which will be discussed below can also lead to heart attack.

UnhealthyLifestyles:

Smoking: Chemicals in cigarette smoke cause the blood to thicken and form clots inside veins and arteries. Blockage from a clot can lead to a heart attack.prolonged inhalation of cigarettes smoke is also harmful to the cardiovascular System.

Prolonged Fumes Inhalation: A large body of science have shown that air pollution can exacerbate existing cardiovascular disease and contribute to the development of the heart disease.Prolonged inhalation of exhaust fumes from generators,trucks, automobiles etc , industrial has pollution can affect the heart system.

Overweight/Obesity: Excess weight can lead to fatty material building up in your arteries (the blood vessels that carry blood to your organs). If the arteries that carry blood to your heart gets damaged and clogged, it can lead to a heart attack.

For overweight individuals,try and loose some pounds/weight, exercise more(gradually but consistently),eat healthy,keep your blood pressure in check and take your pills as prescribed by your doctor.

Excess Sugar: High sugary diets have been linked to high blood pressure, which, in turn, increases the risk of heart disease and stroke. Sugar can promote inflammation in the body which leads to excess stress on the heart and blood vessels.

it's helpful to remember the American Heart Association's recommendations for sugar intake. Men should consume no more than 9 teaspoons (36 grams or 150 calories) of added sugar per day. For women, the number is lower: 6 teaspoons (25 grams or 100 calories) per day.

Lack of Exercise:lack of Execise affects your heart health negatively.When you exercise regularly and moderately,it strengthens your heart muscle. This improves your heart's ability to pump blood to your lungs and throughout your body. As a result, more blood flows to your muscles, and oxygen levels in your blood rises.

Exercise improves oxygen delivery throughout the body.

Physical activity helps control your weight. It also reduces the chances of developing other conditions that may put a strain on the heart, such as high blood pressure, high cholesterol and type 2 diabetes.

The American Heart Association recommends 150 minutes of moderate exercise a week.

Aerobic exercises best for the heart are *Brisk walking, light jogging,swimming, cycling, playing tennis or basketball,yoga ,dancing and more.*

Eating Poorly: A healthy diet can help reduce your risk of developing coronary heart disease and stop you from gaining weight, reducing your risk of diabetes and high blood pressure. It can also help lower your cholesterol levels.Try incorporate more of fruits and veggies in your meal plan.

Late Night Meal: Late-night meals especially with poor choices can lead to increased cholesterol and triglycerides, as well as a higher risk of heart disease and heart attack.

Excess Cold: When you are cold, blood vessels narrow in your skin, fingers and toes, so that less heat is lost. But this narrowing (called 'vasoconstriction') creates more pressure in the rest of the circulation, meaning the heart has to work harder to pump blood around the body, increasing heart rate and blood pressure.Always regulate your Air condition temperature not to be too cold.

Try keep yourself warm especially in cold countries.

Drug Abuse: Wrong drug combinations can trigger blood pressure to rise.If you take medicine to treat high cholesterol, high blood pressure, or diabetes, follow your doctor's instructions carefully.

• Always ask questions if you don't understand something. Never stop taking your medicine without talking to your doctor, nurse, or pharmacist.

Prolonged Absence of Sex

Having sex is good for your heart.Sex is a form of exercise and it helps strengthen your heart and reduce risk of heart disease, lowers your blood pressure, reduce stress and improve sleep.

Poor Sleep: Getting enough quality sleep is an essential component of good heart and brain health. Poor sleep can cause cardiovascular disease risk factors including obesity, <u>high blood pressure</u> and <u>diabetes</u>.

Drinking too much Alcohol: Although light-to-moderate drinking can protect your heart against coronary artery disease. heavy alcohol consumption can damage the cardiovascular system, resulting in maladies such as heart muscle disorders, irregular heart rhythms, high blood pressure, and strokes.

Note:Many drugs, such as cocaine, heroin and various forms of amphetamine, affect the central nervous system and can alter a user's consciousness. In addition to addiction, the side effects and risks associated with use of these drugs include:

. changes in body temperature, heart rate, and blood pressure

- headaches, abdominal pain, and nausea
- impaired judgment and greater risk of some sexually transmitted infections
- the possibility of added substances (such as talc, poisons, herbicides or other particles) which may cause a toxic reaction.
- heart attacks, seizures, and respiratory arrest
- **Always check your Blood pressure at Intervals.**

CONCLUSION

Dietary choices and Lifestyles play an essential role in determining Our Wellbeing over the years. While no single food is a cure-all, consuming a combination of various healthy foods are capable of fending off diseases and also enhance your overall health. Incorporating those heart healthy foods discussed above in your dietary plan alongside a healthy lifestyle will definitely benefit you in the long run. STAY BLESSED.

About the Author.

Antonia Aghaji, B.sc Applied Biochemistry is a Certified health and safety personnel,a health researcher and health enthusiast. As a biochemist,She teaches people on biochemical mechanisms of food in the human body,teaches proper food selections,organic feeding and healthy lifestyles. She's also an interior decorator and a fashion stylist.She's from Anambra State, Nigeria and resides there with her Family.

<u>**To contact Antonia,please send an email to**</u>

<u>**toniaaghaji@gmail.com**</u>

www.ingramcontent.com/pod-product-compliance
Lightning Source LLC
Chambersburg PA
CBHW081807250726
48653CB00010B/3819